THE "7" DAY DETOX | THE 21 DAY GREEN-DETOX FAST

CONGRATULATIONS ON YOUR DECISION TO GET HEALTHY!

THE "7" DAY DETOX | THE 21 DAY GREEN-DETOX FAST

The "7' Day Detox
(The 21 Day Green-Detox Fast)

COOKBOOK II

A guide to a *new eating plan* that is not a "DIET", created based on personal experience to help you *finally* achieve your weight loss and health goals.

ALSO BY KYLA LATRICE, MBA

"New Me, New You! (How I Overcame Obesity)"

"The 7 Day Smoothie Detox"

"The 21 Day Slushie & Juice Fast"

"The 21 Day Salad Fast"

"Eat Well and Stay Thin (Living a Healthy You)"

"21 Days to a New Healthy You! Hearty Vegan & Vegetarian Slow Cooker Recipes"

"Twenty-One Healthy Ice Pop Snack Recipes"

"21 Days of Everyday Healthy Snack Recipes"

"All Natural Soups & Stews"

"A Collection of My Favorite Health Recipes"

"A New You! Workout Workbook"

THE "7" DAY DETOX
The 21 Day Green-Detox Fast

A 21 DAY GREEN-DETOX FAST TO RESET YOUR HEALTH, MIND, BODY, METABOLISM AND *"LIFE"*

KYLA LATRICE, MBA

Lady Mirage Publications, Inc.

New York   Memphis   Los Angeles   London   Cape Town   Toronto
Atlanta   Singapore   Japan

Copyright © 2014 by Ms. Kyla Latrice, Inc.
The author is represented by Lady Mirage Literary Agency, Inc.
All rights reserved. In accordance with the U.S. Copyright Act of 1976, the scanning, uploading, and electronic sharing of any part of this book without the permission of the publisher is unlawful piracy and theft of the author's intellectual property. If you would like to use material from the book (other than for review purposes), prior written permission must be obtained by contacting the publisher at
www.LadyMirageAgency.com
Thank you for your support of the author's rights.

Published by:
Lady Mirage Publications, Inc.
3724 Goodman Rd W, Unit 575
Horn Lake, MS 38637
www.LadyMirageAgency.com

Manufactured in the United States of America
First Edition: July 2014

Lady Mirage Publications, Inc. is an imprint and subsidiary of Lady Mirage Global. The Lady Mirage Publications, Inc. name and logo are trademarks of Lady Mirage Global.

Authors within the Lady Mirage Global (under Lady Mirage Agency, Inc.), Lady Mirage Publications and Lady Mirage Literary Agency speakers division provides a wide range of authors for speaking engagements. To find out more information, go to
www.LadyMirageAgency.com
Cover photo provided by www.FreeDigitalPhotos.net

The publisher is not responsible for websites (or their content) that are not owned by the publisher.

Library of Congress Cataloging-in-Publication Data:
eISBN: 978-1-31-194997-4; Print ISBN: 978-0-9975371-1-6
Tennin, Kyla Latrice.
The "7" Day Detox: The 21 Day Green-Detox Fast
Pages cm; copyrighted materials.
1. Health-Nutrition-Diet-Fitness. 2. Cooking. 3. Fitness.
Library of Congress Catalog Card Number: 2016907244

THE "7" DAY DETOX | THE 21 DAY GREEN-DETOX FAST

Print Book Edition, License Note

This book is licensed for your personal enjoyment only. This book may not be re-sold or given away to other people. If you would like to share this book with another person, please purchase an additional copy for each recipient.
If you're reading this book and did not purchase it, or it was not purchased for your use only, then please return to your favorite book retailer and purchase your own copy. Thank you for respecting the hard work of this author.

Also Note

In this book, Ms. Latrice begins by explaining a *fast* that she has created, tested and tried, which contributed to her weight loss, weight management and healthy eating lifestyle journey. She has also written this book due to there being so many books, health, weight-loss and "diet" programs currently on the global market. The programs and books she has seen and reviewed are too long, too thick, have too much information and many times, are difficult for people to read. This book was written to ***simplify and shorten*** how to lose weight and maintain your health, for life. It is based on personal experience and is still done today. It's an effective solution.

The "7" Day Detox
(The 21 Day Green-Detox Fast)

THE "7" DAY DETOX | THE 21 DAY GREEN-DETOX FAST

Table of Contents

GREEN-DETOX SMOOTHIES..40
Day 1: Apple Carrot Blend...................................42
    Day 2: Carrot Beater…………….…………………44
Day 3: Beat Pear Fix………………………………….46
    Day 4: The Carrot Pruner……………………….…..48
Day 5: Cucumber Apple Finisher……………………..50
    Day 6: The Pineapple Beat Dasher………………..52
Day 7: Pear Carrot Sunriser……………………….54
    Day 8: Pineapple Beat Remix……………………..56
Day 9: Beat Pear Mixer…………………………………58
    Day 10: Apple Carrot Fixer……………………….60
Day 11: Carrot Pruner Repairer………………….…….62
    Day 12: Cucumber Apple Dasher…………….…..64
Day 13: Pear Carrot Remix…………………………66
    Day 14: Carrot Beat Dasher………………...……68
Day 15: The Apple Carrot Lover………………….…..70
    Day 16: Carrot Beat Makeover…………..….……..72
Day 17: Beat Pear Leaner………………………...……74
    Day 18: Carrot Pruner……………………...………76
Day 19: Cucumber Apple Daisy……………….....……78
    Day 20: Pineapple Beat Cleaner…………….……80
Day 21: Pear Carrot Lover……………….….….……82

INDEX…………………………………….……………..84
    Green-Detox Smoothie Recipes…………….84

DEDICATION

This cookbook is dedicated to men and women around the world that have dealt with or are beginning to deal with food addiction, obesity and/or declining health.

I also dedicate this book to those whom have been "Mirage's" in life; overlooked, betrayed, not good enough, slandered, mistreated, misunderstood, misrepresented and even treated unfairly because of their weight or how they looked on the *outside* to others, when in fact, on the *inside* there's greater.

This new cookbook is also dedicated to men and women around the world that want to
shift from being ordinary to extraordinary and accomplishing what others said you would never be able to do again or never be able to do at all.

Here's to the New You!

ACKNOWLEDGMENTS

I want to *say thank you* to anyone whom has ever betrayed, rejected, mistreated, teased, and misused or looked down upon me. You helped me become GREATER and launched me into my destiny.

Whenever someone throws bricks at you, use them to *"build"*. Build something greater; even your mansion.

And whenever you face opposition, "know" that it is actually an opportunity; a set-back for a set-up to secure the victory, rejection for rewards, pain for gain, lack for prosperity to leave a legacy, misery for miracles and put downs for promotion.

IT'S YOUR TIME…*to bounce back!*

Let's Get Healthy!

AUTHOR'S NOTE

"The 7 Day Detox" (The 21 Day Green-Detox Fast)
Copyright © 2014
Ms. Kyla Latrice, Inc.
All Rights Reserved.

AFFIDAVIT

All content written herein is of opinion, from personal experience and of suggestion. Individual smoothie fast and new eating plan results may vary from person to person and no results are guaranteed.

You must put forth effort and do the work necessary to take charge of changing your life and *losing weight*. I did and so can you.

You can also utilize this cookbook if you have already met your weight loss goals and just want to stay healthy with recipes that will keep your metabolism in check and body running smoothly.

Be sure to wash all fruits, vegetables, foods, etc. thoroughly before beginning any new
eating or meal plan.

ALL RIGHTS RESERVED

No portion of this publication may be reproduced, stored in any electronic system, or transmitted in any form by any means; electronic, mechanical,
photocopy, recording or otherwise, without written permission from the author.

Brief quotations may be used in literary reviews with the consent of the author and publisher.

THE "7" DAY DETOX | THE 21 DAY GREEN-DETOX FAST

"ON-THE-GO"

This cookbook *(and all of my cookbooks, books, workbook and manuals)* can be read and applied in airports, on trains, at work on your lunch break, in grocery stores while shopping for and planning your weekly meals, at bookstore cafes, at restaurants *(for quick decision making; to remember your health and/or weight loss goals)* and even in shopping malls.

In addition, *this book can be brought to* fast food restaurants (to pull up and look through to remember your goals before ordering), at the park (before a jog or potluck), during your hotel stays, on vacations and at airport food counters when ordering your meals and drinks *(so you remember your goals and what to eat and drink)*.

This cookbook has been made available on mobile devices via Adobe Digital Editions and DRM (Digital Rights Management).

WORLD STATISTICS

Obesity and Childhood Obesity
Centers for Disease Control and Prevention
http://www.cdc.gov/obesity/data/adult.html
http://www.cdc.gov/nchs/fastats/obesity-overweight.htm

Harvard School of Public Health
http://www.hsph.harvard.edu/obesity-prevention-source/obesity-trends/

World Health Organization
http://www.who.int/topics/obesity/en/

Stroke Awareness and Prevention
http://www.cdc.gov/stroke/facts.htm

Diabetes Awareness and Prevention
Centers for Disease Control and Prevention
http://www.cdc.gov/diabetes/data/statistics/2014statisticsreport.html

American Diabetes Association
http://www.diabetes.org/diabetes-basics/statistics/

THE "7" DAY DETOX | THE 21 DAY GREEN-DETOX FAST

"FASTING"

WHAT IS FASTING?
- Fasting is abstaining from PLEASURABLE foods for a certain amount of time to FOCUS on things that are more important than pleasurable foods to get to the root of what is causing your poor health, obesity, relationships and quality of life.

- It is not a hunger strike.

- You're able to see into your life better and rid it of the bad when you pull away from portion after portion at the dinner table, lunch buffet after buffet with friends and co-workers, nightly binge eating and drinking (whether alcohol, sodas, sugary drinks and the like) and dessert or movie nights on the sofa with a large pizza box and donuts.

- Fasting helps you pinpoint where you overdo things (overindulge), gets you back on track and teaches you how to eat, "in moderation" (balance), for your health and for a better life.

- Your body may not like eating healthy for the first few days (especially if you have never fasted before), but it will adjust.

REASONS FOR FASTING:
- It produces a physical discipline (especially for how, when, where and *what* you eat).

- It rids the body of toxins (just like exercise does when you sweat); cleansing your body and digestive tracts, improving your health and weight.

Note: If you are on medication, consult your physician before any *fast*.

THE "7" DAY DETOX | THE 21 DAY GREEN-DETOX FAST

BENEFITS OF FASTING:

- It strengthens *you* and your body.

- Fasting brings joy, happiness and *energy* to your life; and fruits, vegetables, oils, etc. are quite inexpensive. Make a list and shop for your ingredients before you begin.

- You become very aware of *what* and *how much* you eat. You also begin to pay more attention to when and where you always eat/drink and what leads you to OVEREATING.

- Fasting brings humility, revelation and an overall healthy lifestyle (mind, emotions, intellect, etc.).

TYPICAL TYPES OF FASTS:
Sometimes people fast the following from their lives:
- Television (even the internet, social media or video games) for one day, three days or even one week, television during certain hours of the day (to break a cycle of watching certain shows they may be addicted to (like food) that aren't good for them.

 ….or
- To break a cycle of "certain foods" they may eat while watching certain television shows.

- Fasting to abstain from all pleasurable foods and red meats, eating only fruits, vegetables, clear soups, cereals (no white sugar), water, diluted fruit juices (100% juices only) and/or grains.

- Some people even fast people (bad acquaintances, friendships or relationships), leading eventually to moving away from those person's completely, for a better life and health. Your health is your life.

- Many people fast for 24 hours, three days, seven days, 14 days, 21 days or longer. My success and learning my body as well as other persons bodies (whom have fasted when I have fasted) has come from "closely monitoring" how the body reacts to each of these fasts (particularly "21 days") and I've noticed some things and have sculpted recipes to help others find that tremendous success in many areas of their lives as well.

- Fasts should always be broken slowly, especially if you have been on an "extended fast" (a fast for more than 30 days, a salad only fast, a smoothie only fast or even a clear soup only fast).

- Gradually get back into "regular food", until you can completely commit to "healthy food" (and a regular healthy lifestyle); such as having juices for a couple of days, then fruits, vegetables, grains and adding meats back into your diet last, if applicable.

- Typically, people have six meals per day (three main meals (breakfast, lunch and dinner) and three snacks). For each of my Fasts or Recipes, you determine how many meals. Don't worry, fruits and vegetables do not cause obesity, they prevent it. Yet, always watch your portion sizes, in general, and with soups, stews and anything that has meat included. Never eat meat in excess.

- You can even choose to eat one meal per day for 21 days (there are enough recipes listed in this book), a snack, have 5-8 bottles of water and be sure to get a nap in and some exercise during the week. As you advance you can mix your salad fast with a smoothie fast and detox fast by doing one of the fasts, each per week, for 21 days, etc.

THE "7" DAY DETOX | THE 21 DAY GREEN-DETOX FAST

THE *"GREEN-DETOX FAST"* BIRTH

Kyla Latrice is a native of Marks, MS and enjoys food and traveling. Being from a small town and a country gal, she set her goals high. Graduating from a private institution with a Bachelor of Arts Degree (BA) *(women's studies and health background; pre-medicine)* and a Master's Degree (MBA) in Business Administration with **Executive Education at Harvard and Stanford** along with several certifications and nearly 50-80 self-study coursework in legal, intellectual property and self-help, she has become one of the leading entrepreneurs of her time.

Currently Ms. Latrice is finishing up her Doctoral Honorary Degree *(**Doctor of Management in Organizational Leadership**)* and continues to serve on Board of Directors throughout the world for various causes; still relating to her life's purpose and corporations work. Ms. Latrice travels extensively for speaking engagements in the areas of health, wellness, obesity, poverty, domestic violence, branding, image, leadership, mentoring, business, entrepreneurship and the like.

To date, Ms. Latrice has mentored with over 20 plus organizations *(from elementary to senior citizen)*, helping others overcome issues she has faced.

With her first *corporate* job opportunity being at a "Health Food Restaurant" *(when she was age 15 or 16)* to work as a deli attendant at the deli bar, hostess *(when others were out for the day)* and bakery attendant as well as a chef in the *salad bar*.

Her main role was to attend to the deli, to prepare healthy pasta salads, healthy sandwiches, healthy shakes, healthy sundaes and *healthy smoothies*. However, Ms. Latrice was blessed with the opportunity to be called upon whenever management needed her help in the other areas as well, **to continue learning**. This gave Ms. Latrice very valuable experience and a "look" into health and business ownership, a bit deeper, which still remains with her today.

THE *"GREEN-DETOX FAST"* BIRTH

KYLA LATRICE
BEFORE
21 DAY GREEN-DETOX FASTS

Ms. Latrice's *(on the left in the photo)* Corporations are inclusive of health restaurants, retail stores, property and land as well as product development organizations along with nonprofit foundations to care for the displaced, homeless.

Further, Ms. Latrice's love for food turned into obesity when her life took a turn in the early 2000's during domestic violence, sinful relationships, bad friendships, emotional binge eating and more; then again in the 2000's with another domestic violence relationship, obesity slander from family members, mental and spiritual abuse, abortion, home foreclosure, vehicle repossession and much *more*, which all have an effect on health, but she made sure her Corporations still stood; to help others.

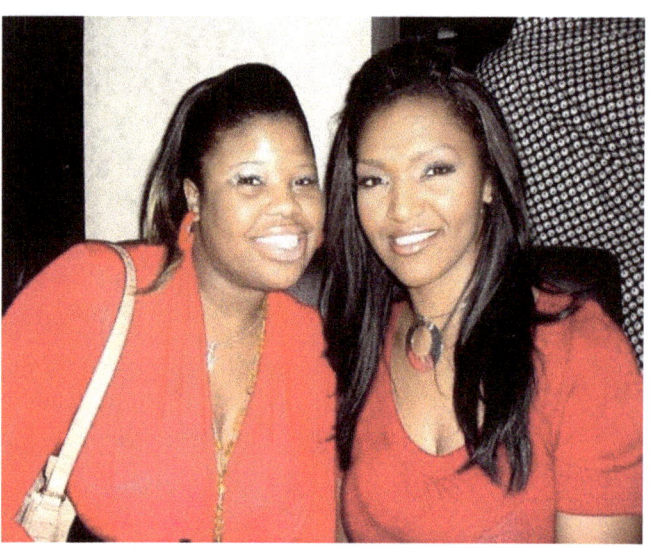

THE *"GREEN-DETOX FAST"*
BIRTH

KYLA LATRICE
"IN THE MIDDLE"
AFTER GAINING WEIGHT BACK FOR A SECOND TIME
21 DAY GREEN-DETOX FASTS

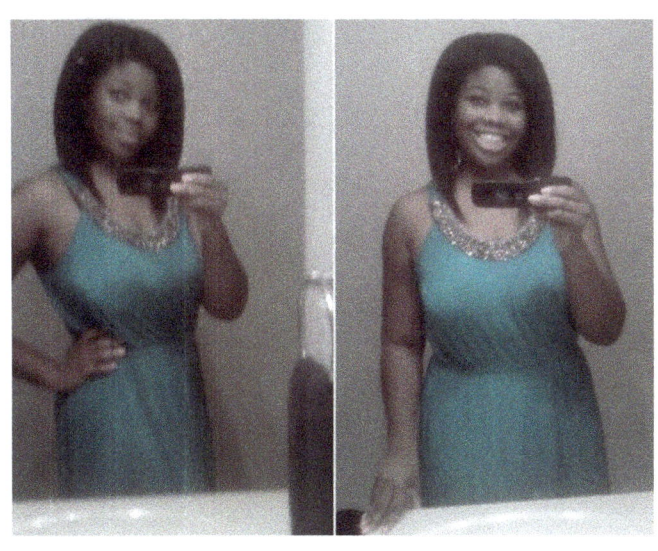

THE *"GREEN-DETOX FAST"* BIRTH

KYLA LATRICE
AFTER
21 DAY GREEN-DETOX FASTS

THE FINALE

THE "7" DAY DETOX | THE 21 DAY GREEN-DETOX FAST

Many factors can contribute to obesity, such as abuse *(mental, spiritual, physical, sexual)*, poor eating habits, environment, bad friendships, sin and more. Personally, I, myself, was never taught how to eat, I did not know what to eat *(that was truly healthy for me)* and I did not know how to deal with life's problems.

Nevertheless, how can someone teach you what they don't know? My first encounter with obesity was when I was a model and went from a size 0 to a size 20/22, **weighing close to 300 pounds** *(then I lost nearly 115 pounds after prayer and seeking a remedy)*.

The second encounter was when I gained some of the first encounters weight back and went from a size 14/16 to a size 4/6 and fitting a 7/8 in jeans, losing 68 pounds. Today, I am going to share my secrets to success with you *(the birth of the "21 Day Salad Fast")* and how I made it out over the years **and** kept the weight off. Let's get started and healthy, for life!

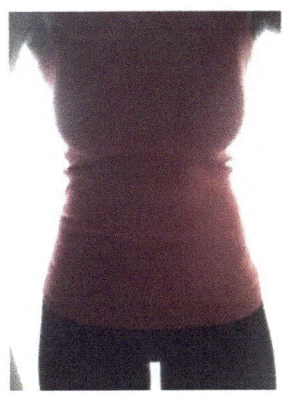
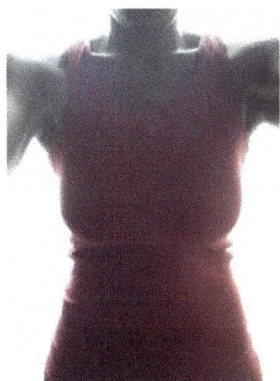

GETTING HEALTHY
LIFESTYLE CHANGE

THE "7" DAY DETOX | THE 21 DAY GREEN-DETOX FAST

Prepare to lose weight on the "Detox Fast" (this is not a "diet", this is an "eating plan" to reprogram your mind, body and metabolism about how to eat (portion control) and regarding what foods you should and should not be eating). It is designed to help you become healthier. Before starting this fast and any of my eating *plans ("The 21 Day Smoothie Fast" and "The 21 Day Salad Fast" as well as "Soups and Stews")*, allow yourself "one week" to prepare for the fast and eating plan by removing the following from your life:

➢ Negative relationships and friendships; they block you from doing well in life and succeeding, when people begin to see you doing well, they tend to not like it. Choose friendships and associations wisely. Be creative.

➢ Bad acquaintances; they will eventually want what you have and will cause betrayal to take place in your life through a "set-up" to sabotage all of your hard work. Always keep moving forward.

➢ Remove the following (slowly) from your daily meals (eating habits) because they contribute to weight gain (some quicker than others): soda, breads, pastas, candy bars and the like and eating second, third and fourth portions of your food. You only need one portion. Don't eat the rest!

➢ Replace all sodas with diet soda until you can cut soda out of your daily meal plan completely; only drink soda if absolutely necessary *(a lemon-lime beverage)* because there is nothing else to drink. For example, while traveling.

➢ Remove all "junk food" (cakes, pies, chips, all kinds of desserts and the like) from your kitchen.

- For breads, certain kinds make the weight gain skyrocket; be careful about pizza. Pasta should be limited just like soda, having it only if absolutely necessary, but once every 2-4 months is okay, just like donuts, to stay **balanced** and give your body a break from always eating healthy.

- Again, you only need one portion of food, per meal, work on this and you'll see results quicker.

- Increase your water intake to 5-8 bottled waters a day; bring a bottle with you everywhere you go so you'll be forced to drink it *(instead of something else)* and will program your body to like it *(whether you like it frozen, warm or cold)*.

- When you're out to eating with others, begin selecting items from menus that help *(not hinder)* your **new eating plan**, for example, order a "grilled chicken wrap with a side salad and small water" instead of a double cheeseburger, french fries and large soda. Never super-size, it wastes your results and time spent on improving your health.

- If you have not already, purchase my books: *"The 21 Day Smoothie Fast"* and *"The 21 Day Salad Fast"* to begin, to continue your weight loss and new you.

- And again, remember, commit to single portion eating, eating smaller portions (always have more vegetables on your plate than poultry/ meat), and increase your water intake *(remember to use the restroom)*. Let's begin.

THE "7" DAY DETOX | THE 21 DAY GREEN-DETOX FAST

GETTING HEALTHY
SET GOALS

Feel free to purchase my "A New Healthy You Workout Workbook" *(to go with your **new eating plan** and my "fasts" cookbooks* or a composition notebook from any retailer to make your own journal to measure the following (even if you need to do so at your primary care physician's office, a free clinic or go to a free health assessment machine in a retail store location that has one):

Record a written record of each:

- Your Cholesterol Level.
- Blood Pressure and Vision Check.
- Your actual Height Weight, Height, Bust/Chest and Hips size (write down your goals of where you want to be in the next week, three months, six months and year).
- Record your weight, chest/bust, hips and waist size every Saturday morning at 7am.
- Stroll through a department store and notate clothing (or take a camera phone photo) you plan on fitting into someday and notate your current sizes and then return in three months to see how you're fairing up towards your goals.
- Pick up my *"A New Healthy You Workout Workbook"* or list in your journal, your reasons for losing weight, changing your life and changing your eating habits.

THE "7" DAY DETOX | THE 21 DAY GREEN-DETOX FAST

- Your BMI (Body Mass Index) and where you are versus where you're supposed to be for your height, weight, age and gender.
- Bottles of "cold water" listed in the recipes section of this book are in reference to drinking 4-5 bottles of 16 fl oz bottles of water, which is equivalent to 8-10 glasses of water per day.
- Water is vital for living and for being healthy.
- The amount of water within the human body is typically 50-65% water and in infants, 78%.
- Water assists your body with digesting food and getting nutrients from the foods you have eaten to your blood, brain and other parts of your body, in order to function; emptying the body of waste and toxins, helps deliver oxygen to the body, helps prevent constipation and even regulates body temperature (in your cells, organs and tissues).

A (BMI) Chart is below for your convenience.

BMI	<(less than) 18.5	=	Underweight
BMI	18.5-24.9	=	Normal Weight
BMI	25-29.9	=	Overweight
BMI	>(more than) 30	=	Obese

GETTING HEALTHY
WHILE TRAVELING

THE "7" DAY DETOX | THE 21 DAY GREEN-DETOX FAST

If you'll be traveling by airplane, helicopter or private jet (smile):

- Research where you will be eating ahead of time (food choices, ingredients and prices).
- Bring bottled water.
- Resist vending machines and relying of fast food at your final destination.
- Bring your own snacks (trail mix, cashews, a banana, apple slices, peanuts) and
- Workout for free in your hotel room, taking the stairs instead of elevators and walking at the Mall.

If traveling by car:

- Pack your own cooler with ice for your bottled waters, fruits and raw vegetables.
- Consider bringing a bag of oranges & any other food that can be eaten warm or cold on the road.

If you'll be traveling by bus, train, or other means:

- Research where you will be eating ahead of time (food choices, ingredients and prices).
- Bring bottled water.
- Bring your own snacks (trail mix, cashews, a banana, apple slices, peanuts for the long trip) and
- Bring something to read or play, to keep your mind off of food and *fictious* hunger.
- At your destination, stand more than you sit (to keep your body moving) and since you have been sitting during traveling for your trip.

SPINACH

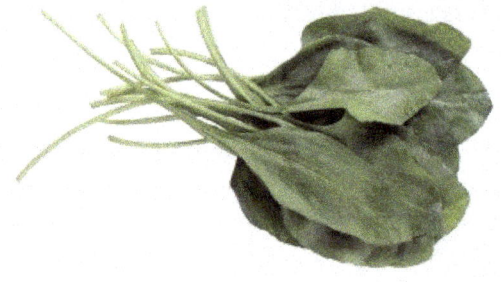

Photo Credit: Smarnad
Freedigitalphotos.net

THE "7" DAY DETOX | THE 21 DAY GREEN-DETOX FAST

GETTING HEALTHY
YOUR NEW WORKOUT PLAN

During my both times of being obese, I never worked out at a gym nor went outside of my home to run *(weighing in at 278 pounds and trying to start my "new me" as a jogger was terrible on my knees)* to lose weight, I did it all at home, on the floor, in a compact room, near a closet. I suggest you begin a "workout regime" by doing simple workouts, such as crunches, stretching, leg lifts and a few push-ups.

Everyone cannot do cardio in the gym (paid membership prices or because of lack of transportation), running outside or bouncing around in-doors for 1-3 hours like actors and actresses on television, whom are likely being *paid monetary* compensation or by other means to film the infomercial.

Remain constant and do this 3-4 times a week, for 15-35 minutes each day. On your workout OFF days, do 100 crunches before going to bed. Consider purchasing my "Workout Workbook" to keep up with your Fitness Plan. In addition, you burn calories when you sleep, by drinking water, by exercising (which helps you live longer as well) and by **movement** (whether your arms, legs, looking out of a window, etc.).

Furthermore, water helps break down food and helps food digest. Your can also do a "mental workout" by cutting out negative people, places and things from your life.

You'll find that you have more peace in your brain and life, when you replace them with reading inspirational books, movies, community work and exercise or things you love, such as knitting, a ball game, taking a site seeing road trip (alone) every now and then or mentoring someone.

THE "7" DAY DETOX | THE 21 DAY GREEN-DETOX FAST

Notes

THE SIX MONTH RULE
GIVE IT *"TIME"*

THE SIX-MONTH RULE
On a 21-Day Detox Fast, weight [pounds] have been known to drop quickly for many people. However, the goal here is to also keep the weight off. Stay focused and be committed to at least six-months of "health work".

Remember to journal your progress.

There's something about when you write things down, they get *ACCOMPLISHED!* Also give yourself a total of six-months to work on your "New You" simply because you may lose inches first and not weight, until your weight catches up with your inches (this is what took place with me; loosing 10-12 pounds per month).

Inches first then one day the weight just fell off. And for others, sometimes weight first, then inches.

GO BACK TO THE DEPARTMENT STORE
Revisit those same department stores that you went to on the first week of your new lifestyle change, try on new clothing sizes to see where you are with your goals.

I suggest that you "mentally shop" for a new suit, a dinner dress, clothing for you next vacation (Hawaii maybe), your first pair of skinny jeans or baseball gear to wear to a game; all after you have reached your goals; to *CELEBRATE!*

"GREEN-DETOX"
RECIPES

THE "7" DAY DETOX | THE 21 DAY GREEN-DETOX FAST

WEEK 1
SPINACH WEEK

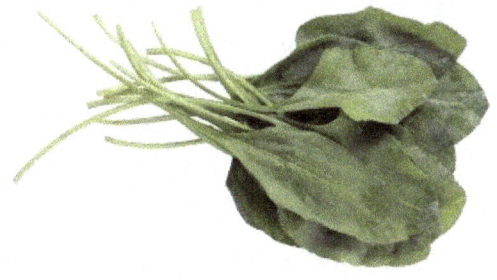

Photo Credit: Smarnad
Freedigitalphotos.net

WEEK 1, DAY 1
(THE APPLE CARROT BLEND)

Day 1 of Week 1: Apple, Carrot, 100% Vegetable Juice

Add 1 cup of a diced yellow apple (not green) into a blender, Add 1 cup of a diced carrot, Add 1/2 cup of 100% Vegetable Juice, Add 1/2 cup of spinach, blend until smooth, pour into a chilled glass or bullet to go blender cup or blender mug, Serve immediately

Health Notes:

Apples – Apples help whiten your teeth by producing saliva, assisting with reducing tooth decay, protects against cancers, gallstones, hemorrhoids, constipation and high cholesterol. They also help you control your weight, prevent cataracts, decrease your chances of developing diabetes and boost your immune system (red apples; which have an antioxidant called quercetin in them). Apples also have Vitamins C, A and Flavonoids, Phosphorus, Iron and Calcium as well as Potassium to help promote heart health.

Carrots - Carrots can be white, yellow, red, purple and orange. They are also great for your teeth, killing off harmful germs in the mouth to help prevent tooth decay. Carrots also have a great source of Vitamins A, beta carotene *(an antioxidant to help maintain healthy skin),* Alkaline elements (which help purify and revitalize the blood) and Potassium *(helping the body maintain normal blood pressure levels).*

Spinach – Spinach are filled with Vitamins C, E, beta-carotene and even zinc. They also have a large amount of Vitamin K *(helping with brain function)* helping the nervous system and fighting stroke and cardiovascular disease. Spinach also help prevent osteoporosis, high blood pressure, vision problems and immune deficiencies *(such as intestinal tract infections).*

Weight Loss Tip: Drink 4-5 bottles of cold water today.

THE "7" DAY DETOX | THE 21 DAY GREEN-DETOX FAST

CARROTS

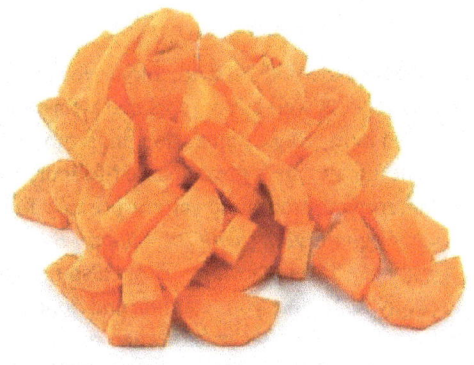

Photo Credit: Grant Cochrane
Freedigitalphotos.net

WEEK 1, DAY 2
(CARROT BEATER)

Day 2 of Week 1: Carrot, Beat, 100% Vegetable Juice, Shot of Wheatgrass, Spinach

Add 1 cup of a diced carrot into a blender, Add 1 cup of a diced beat, Add 1 small cup of juiced (or non-juiced) wheatgrass, Add 1/2 cup of 100% Vegetable Juice, , Add 1/2 cup of spinach, blend until smooth, pour into a chilled glass or bullet to go blender cup or blender mug, Serve immediately

Health Notes:

Beats – Beats cleanse the body and are a tonic for the liver and purifies the blood as well as prevents many forms of cancer. Beats also help reduce depression, high blood pressure, give energy and are a great source of Fiber, Vitamins A, B & C, beta-carotene, Iron, folic acid *(especially for women that are pregnant along with the Vitamin B and Iron)* as well as Potassium and Magnesium. Beats also help you detoxify your body and boost your stamina and bone strength and help fight Alzheimer's disease and inflammation.

Wheatgrass – Wheatgrass is rich in Calcium, Iron, Vitamins A and E and Chlorophyll (helping build the blood). Wheatgrass also stimulates circulation of oxygen in your body, blood vessels and skin and rids your body of waste. It also helps prevent cancers and tooth decay as well as treats wounds, fatigue, arthritis, sunburn, ulcers (improving digestion), dryness or eczema of the skin (discoloration) and cleanses the skin and liver.

Weight Loss Tip: Drink 4-5 bottles of cold water today.

THE "7" DAY DETOX | THE 21 DAY GREEN-DETOX FAST

BEATS

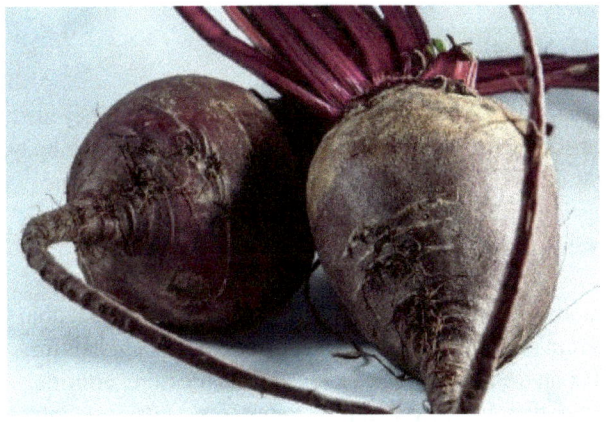

Photo Credit: digidreamgrafix
Freedigitalphotos.net

WEEK 1, DAY 3
(BEAT PEAR FIX)

Day 3 of Week 1: Beat, Pear, dash of squeezed lemon, 100% Vegetable Juice, Spinach

Add 1 cup of a diced beat into a blender, Add 1 cup of a diced pear, Add 1/2 of a squeezed lemon, Add 1/2 cup of 100% Vegetable Juice, Add 1/2 cup of spinach, blend until smooth, pour into a chilled glass or bullet to go blender cup or blender mug, Serve immediately

Health Notes:

Pears – Pears are filled with Vitamin C and Iron. They are a great source of fiber; help reduce bad cholesterol in the body, fights cancer, acne and aging, increases energy levels and digestion. Pears also help restore shine to your hair and prevents frizz.

Lemons – Lemons are a great source of citric acid, Vitamin C, Calcium and even Potassium. They also help fight hair loss, lumps on the skin and hands, high blood pressure, arthritis, constipation, burns, vision loss, excess gas, gallstones, internal bleeding, fevers and indigestion and aids in cleansing the teeth & dandruff from the hair.

Spinach – Spinach are filled with Vitamins C, E, beta-carotene and even zinc. They also have a large amount of Vitamin K *(helping with brain function)* helping the nervous system and fighting stroke and cardiovascular disease.

Weight Loss Tip: Drink 4-5 bottles of cold water today.

THE "7" DAY DETOX | THE 21 DAY GREEN-DETOX FAST

LEMONS

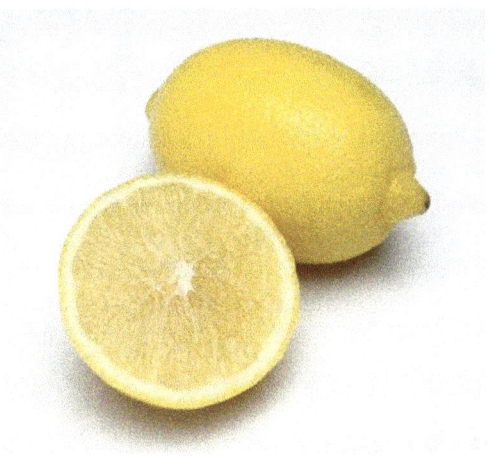

Photo Credit: Suat Eman
Freedigitalphotos.net

WEEK1, DAY 4
(THE CARROT PRUNER)

Day 4 of Week 1: Carrot, Prune, 100% Vegetable Juice, Spinach (in the middle of the week to clean bowels)

Add 1 cup of a diced carrot into a blender, Add a squeeze of fresh lemon juice, Add 1 cup of a diced prune, Add 1/2 cup of 100% Vegetable Juice, Add 1/2 cup of spinach, blend until smooth, pour into a chilled glass or bullet to go blender cup or blender mug, Serve immediately

Health Notes:

Prunes – Prunes aid in weight loss by assisting with bowel movement and relieving constipation. Constipation is also accompanied by bloating, stomach cramps, appetite loss and even headache symptoms. Prunes also are rich in Fiber, Vitamins C and A, boosting your immune system and protecting the heart, fighting against Osteoporosis (a reduction in bone mass). These beauties also fight against cancers, obesity and diabetes.

Spinach – Spinach are filled with Vitamins C, E, beta-carotene and even zinc. They also have a large amount of Vitamin K *(helping with brain function)* helping the nervous system and fighting stroke and cardiovascular disease. Spinach also help prevent osteoporosis, high blood pressure, vision problems *(protecting the eyes from cataracts and macular degeneration as you age)* and immune deficiencies *(such as urinary, respiratory and intestinal tract infections; strengthening these tracts).*

Weight Loss Tip: Drink 4-5 bottles of cold water today.

THE "7" DAY DETOX | THE 21 DAY GREEN-DETOX FAST

CUCUMBERS

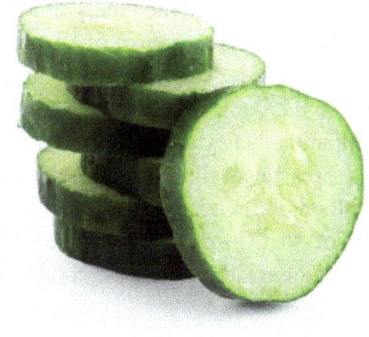

Photo Credit: SOMMAI
Freedigitalphotos.net

WEEK 1, DAY 5
(THE CUCUMBER APPLE FINISHER)

Day 5 of Week 1: Cucumber, Apple, 100% Vegetable Juice, Spirulina, Spinach

Add 1 cup of a 1/2 diced cucumber into a blender, Add 1 cup of a diced yellow apple (not green), Add 1/2 cup of 100% Vegetable Juice, Add a small amount of Spirulina, Add 1/2 cup of spinach, blend until smooth, pour into a chilled glass or bullet to go blender cup or blender mug, Serve immediately

Health Notes:

Cucumbers – Cucumbers are in the family of melons, squash and pumpkins. They are a great source of Vitamins K, C, A and B and are made up 95% water and are great for the eyes, skin and hair due to their anti-inflammatory properties and hair growth stimulation. They also help fight cancers (ovarian, uterine, breast as well as prostate) and aid in weight loss, digestion, blood pressure control, cholesterol reduction and joint pain relief (that is associated with arthritis). Cucumbers also dissolve kidney stones and rid the body of waste products.

Spirulina – Spirulina is a natural algae powder that is rich in B-12 and high in protein. It is also rich in iron, zinc, copper, magnesium, selenium, potassium, Vitamins B-2 (riboflavin), B-3 (nicotinamide), B-9 (folic acid), Omega 3, Omega 9 and Omega 6, Vitamins C, E, A and D as well as B-1 (thiamine) to name a few. Spirulina increases fat burning during exercise, aids in weight loss, removing toxins from the body, inflammatory reduction protects the liver from damage and boosts energy.

Weight Loss Tip: Drink 4-5 bottles of cold water today.

PINEAPPLE

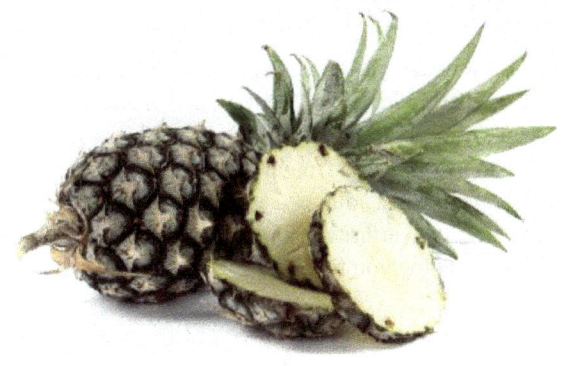

Photo Credit: Rakratchada Torsap
Freedigitalphotos.net

WEEK 1, DAY 6
(THE PINEAPPLE BEAT DASHER)

Day 6 of Week 1: Pineapple, Beat, dash of squeezed lemon, 100% Vegetable Juice, Spinach

Add 1 cup of a diced pineapple into a blender, Add 1 cup of a diced beat, Add a squeezed lemon juice from a 1/2 of a lemon, Add 1/2 cup of 100% Vegetable Juice, Add 1/2 cup of spinach, blend until smooth, pour into a chilled glass or bullet to go blender cup or blender mug, Serve immediately

Health Notes:

Pineapples – Today, the largest producers of pineapples are in Brazil, Costa Rica, the United States, Hawaii and the Philippines. Pineapples are a natural weight loss food and are rich in Vitamin C, Thiamin, copper and boost the immune system to fight against colds, flu symptoms and other diseases. They also help ease arthritis pain, are low in calories and are very filling; keeping you fuller longer, to prevent overeating.

Lemons – Lemons are a great source of citric acid, Vitamin C, Calcium and even Potassium. They also help fight hair loss, lumps on the skin and hands, high blood pressure, arthritis, constipation, burns, vision loss, excess gas, gallstones, internal bleeding, fevers and indigestion as well as aids in cleansing the teeth and dandruff from the hair. Lemons also help revitalize your skin and aid in weight loss when mixed with recipes that have water (or ice) and honey in them.

Weight Loss Tip: Drink 4-5 bottles of cold water today.

PEARS

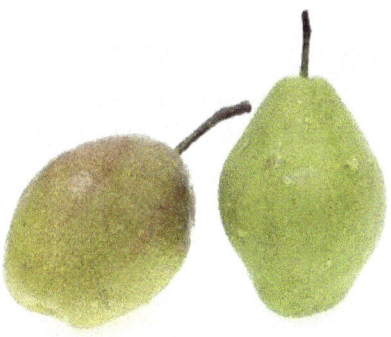

Photo Credit: PhasinPhoto
Freedigitalphotos.net

WEEK 1, DAY 7
(THE PEAR CARROT SUNRISER)
Day 7 of Week 1: Pear, Carrot, 100% Vegetable Juice, Spinach

Add 1 cup of a diced pear into a blender, Add 1 cup of a diced carrot, Add 1/2 cup of 100% Vegetable Juice, Add 1/2 cup of spinach, blend until smooth, pour into a chilled glass or bullet to go blender cup or blender mug, Serve immediately

==Health Notes:==

Pears – Pears are filled with Vitamin C and Iron. They are a great source of fiber; help reduce bad cholesterol in the body, fights cancer, acne and aging, increases energy levels and digestion. Pears also help restore shine to your hair and prevents frizz.

Spinach – Spinach are filled with Vitamins C, E, beta-carotene and even zinc. They also have a large amount of Vitamin K *(helping with brain function)* helping the nervous system and fighting stroke and cardiovascular disease. They also help maintain strong bones and prevent excess activation of osteoclasts (cells that break down bones).

Spinach also help prevent osteoporosis, high blood pressure, vision problems *(protecting the eyes from cataracts and macular degeneration as you age)* and immune deficiencies *(such as urinary, respiratory and intestinal tract infections; strengthening these tracts)*.

Weight Loss Tip: Drink 4-5 bottles of cold water today.

WEEK 2
PARSLEY & KALE WEEK

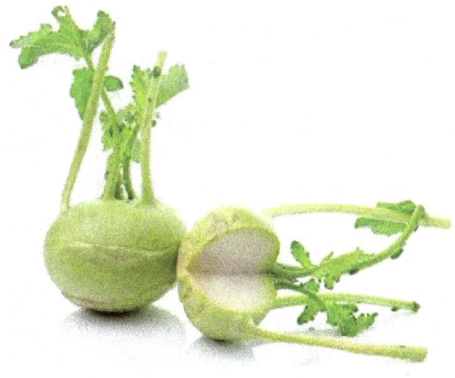

Photo Credit: SOMMAI
Freedigitalphotos.net

WEEK 2, DAY 8
(PINEAPPLE BEAT REMIX)

Day 1 of Week 2: Pineapple, Beat, 100% Carrot Juice, Parsley, Kale

Add 1 cup of a diced pineapple into a blender, Add 1 cup of a diced beat, Add 1/2 cup of 100% Carrot Juice, Add 1/2 cup of parsley, Add 1/2 cup of kale, blend until smooth, pour into a chilled glass or bullet to go blender cup or blender mug, Serve immediately

Health Notes:

Carrots - Carrots can be white, yellow, red, purple and orange. They are also great for your teeth, killing off harmful germs in the mouth to help prevent tooth decay.

Kale – Kale aids in detoxifying the body and in weight loss (digestion). One cup of Kale has zero fat and is extremely low in calories. It increases your metabolism and is rich in Vitamins A, C, K, Folic Acid, B-6 *(preventing heart disease)* and Fiber as well as Omega 3 and Omega 6 for healthy skin, nails, hair, immune system, a clean liver and fights disease and cancers.

Parsley - Parsley comes from the Mediterranean and is rich in Folic Acid, Vitamins C, K, B-12 and A. Parsley boots your immune system (for healthy bones and teeth and preventing urinary, respiratory and intestinal tract infections, excess gas, asthma, diabetes and kidney stones), helps build strong bones, flushes excess fluid from your kidneys, bladder and body, while helping reduce hair loss, high blood pressure, joint pain, constipation, helps fight illness, cancers *(breast and prostate)* and spleen conditions.

Weight Loss Tip: Drink 4-5 bottles of cold water today.

PEARS

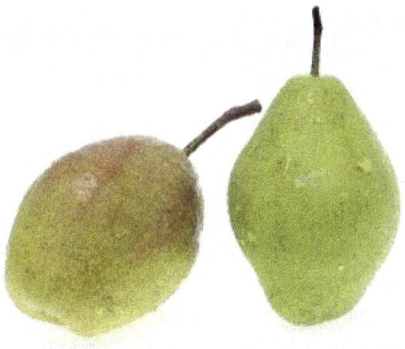

Photo Credit: PhasinPhoto
Freedigitalphotos.net

WEEK 2, DAY 9
(BEAT PEAR MIXER)

Day 2 of Week 2: Beat, Pear, 100% Carrot Juice, Ginseng, Parsley, Kale

Add 1 cup of a diced beat into a blender, Add 1 cup of a diced pear, Add 1/2 cup of 100% Carrot Juice, Add 1/2 cup of parsley, Add a small piece of ginseng, Add 1/2 cup of kale, blend until smooth, pour into a chilled glass or bullet to go blender cup or blender mug, Serve immediately

==Health Notes:==

Pears – Pears are filled with Vitamin C and Iron. They are a great source of fiber; help reduce bad cholesterol in the body, fights cancer, acne and aging, increases energy levels and digestion. Pears also help restore shine to your hair and prevents frizz.

Ginseng – Ginseng comes in Asian, Korean or American. Ginseng helps improve mood and helps fight fatigue, cancers, heart disease, hepatitis C, menopausal systems and high blood sugar levels. Ginseng also boosts energy, concentration and learning. It also helps slow the signs of aging, reduces stress and menstrual cramps, aids in weight loss (fighting obesity) and fights diabetes.

Kale – Kale aids in detoxifying the body and in weight loss (digestion). One cup of Kale has zero fat and is extremely low in calories. It increases your metabolism and is rich in Vitamins A, C, K, Folic Acid, B-6 *(preventing heart disease)* and Fiber as well as Omega 3 and Omega 6 for healthy skin, nails, hair, immune system, a clean liver and fights disease and cancers.

Weight Loss Tip: Drink 4-5 bottles of cold water today.

CARROTS

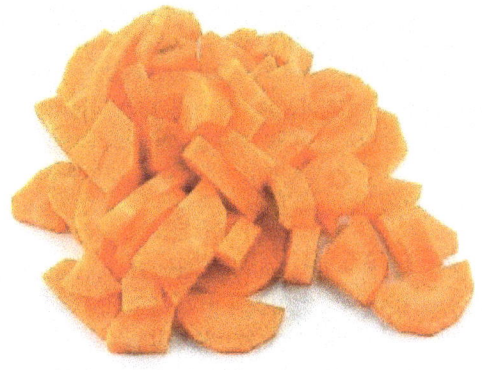

Photo Credit: Grant Cochrane
Freedigitalphotos.net

WEEK 2, DAY 10
(APPLE CARROT FIXER)

Day 3 of Week 2: Apple, Carrot, dash of squeezed lime, 100% Carrot Juice, Parsley, Kale

Add 1 cup of a diced yellow apple (not green) into a blender, Add 1 cup of a diced carrot, squeezed lime, Add 1/2 cup of 100% Carrot Juice, Add 1/2 cup of parsley, Add 1/2 cup of kale, blend until smooth, pour into a chilled glass or bullet to go blender cup or blender mug, Serve immediately

Health Notes:

Apples – Apples help whiten your teeth by producing saliva, assisting with reducing tooth decay, protects against cancers, gallstones, hemorrhoids, constipation and high cholesterol. They also help you control your weight, prevent cataracts, decrease your chances of developing diabetes and boost your immune system (red apples; which have an antioxidant called quercetin in them).

Limes – Limes are rich in Vitamin C and folate. Interestingly, you may think, the juice, fruit and peel of a lime are used to make medicines and help cure severe diarrhea. Limes also kill germs in the skin, aiding in skin care *(preventing aging);* they ease constipation and help prevent fever, urinary tract and bladder infections, ulcers, heart disease *(lowering bad cholesterol)* and even arthritis.

Kale – Kale aids in detoxifying the body and in weight loss (digestion). One cup of Kale has zero fast and is extremely low in calories. It increases your metabolism and is rich in Vitamins A, C, K, Folic Acid, B-6 *(preventing heart disease)* and Fiber as well as Omega 3 and Omega 6 for healthy skin, nails, hair, immune system, a clean liver and fights disease and cancers.

Weight Loss Tip: Drink 4-5 bottles of cold water today.

THE "7" DAY DETOX | THE 21 DAY GREEN-DETOX FAST

APPLES

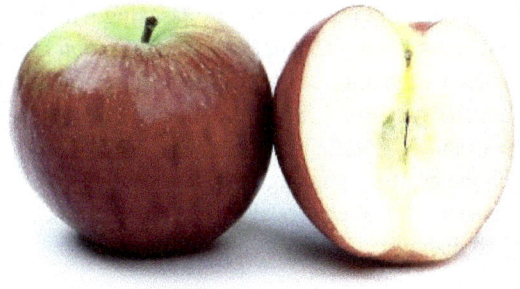

Photo Credit: Paul
Freedigitalphotos.net

WEEK 2, DAY 11
(CARROT PRUNER REPAIRER)

Day 4 of Week 2: Carrot, Prune, 100% Carrot Juice, Parsley, Kale (in the middle of the week to clean bowels)

Add 1 cup of a diced carrot into a blender, Add 1/2 cup of a parsley, Add ½ cup of Kale, Add 1 cup of a diced Apple, Add 1/2 cup of 100% Carrot Juice, Add 1/2 cup of dice prunes, blend until smooth, pour into a chilled glass or bullet to go blender cup or blender mug, Serve immediately

Health Notes:

Prunes – Prunes aid in weight loss by assisting with bowel movement and relieving constipation. Constipation is also accompanied by bloating, stomach cramps, appetite loss and even headache symptoms. Prunes also are rich in Fiber, Vitamins C and A, boosting your immune system and protecting the heart, fighting against Osteoporosis (a reduction in bone mass). These beauties also fight against cancers, obesity and diabetes.

Parsley - Parsley comes from the Mediterranean and is rich in Folic Acid, Vitamins C, K, B-12 and A. Parsley boots your immune system (for healthy bones and teeth and preventing urinary, respiratory and intestinal tract infections, excess gas, asthma, diabetes and kidney stones), helps build strong bones, flushes excess fluid from your kidneys, bladder and body, while helping reduce hair loss, high blood pressure, joint pain, constipation, helps fight illness, cancers *(breast and prostate)* and spleen conditions.

Weight Loss Tip: Drink 4-5 bottles of cold water today.

CUCUMBERS

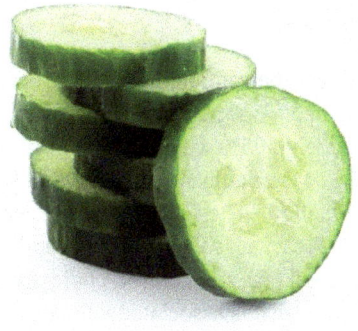

Photo Credit: SOMMAI
Freedigitalphotos.net

WEEK 2, DAY 12
(CUCUMBER APPLE DASHER)

Day 5 of Week 2: Cucumber, Apple, 100% Carrot Juice, Shot of Wheatgrass, Kale

Add 1 cup of a 1/2 diced cucumber into a blender, Add 1 cup of a diced apple, Add 1 small cup of juiced (or non-juiced) wheatgrass, Add 1/2 cup of 100% Carrot Juice, Add 1/2 cup of parsley, Add 1/2 cup of kale, blend until smooth, pour into a chilled glass or bullet to go blender cup or blender mug, Serve immediately

Health Notes:

Cucumbers – Cucumbers are in the family of melons, squash and pumpkins. They are a great source of Vitamins K, C, A and B and are made up 95% water and are great for the eyes, skin and hair due to their anti-inflammatory properties and hair growth stimulation. They also help fight cancers (ovarian, uterine, breast as well as prostate) and aid in weight loss, digestion, blood pressure control, cholesterol reduction and joint pain relief (that is associated with arthritis).

Kale – Kale aids in detoxifying the body and in weight loss (digestion). One cup of Kale has zero fat and is extremely low in calories. It increases your metabolism and is rich in Vitamins A, C, K, Folic Acid, B-6 *(preventing heart disease)* and Fiber as well as Omega 3 and Omega 6 for healthy skin, nails, hair, immune system, a clean liver and fights disease and cancers.

Weight Loss Tip: Drink 4-5 bottles of cold water today.

LIMES

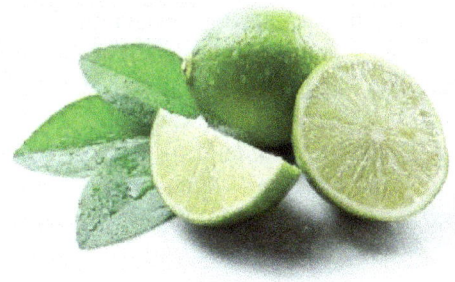

Photo Credit: Master Isolated Images
Freedigitalphotos.net

WEEK 2, DAY 13
(PEAR CARROT REMIX)

Day 6 of Week 2: Pear, Carrot, dash of squeezed lime, 100% Carrot Juice, Parsley, Kale

Add 1 cup of a diced pear into a blender, Add 1 cup of a diced carrot, Add 1/2 cup of 100% Carrot Juice, Add a dash of squeezed lime, Add 1/2 cup of parsley, Add 1/2 cup of kale, blend until smooth, pour into a chilled glass or bullet to go blender cup or blender mug, Serve immediately

Health Notes:

Carrots - Carrots can be white, yellow, red, purple and orange. They are also great for your teeth, killing off harmful germs in the mouth to help prevent tooth decay. Carrots also have a great source of Vitamin A, beta carotene *(an antioxidant to help maintain healthy skin),* Alkaline elements (which help purify and revitalize the blood) and Potassium *(helping the body maintain normal blood pressure levels).*

Pears – Pears are filled with Vitamin C and Iron. They are a great source of fiber; help reduce bad cholesterol in the body, fights cancer, acne and aging, increases energy levels and digestion. Pears also help restore shine to your hair and prevents frizz.

Limes – Limes are rich in Vitamin C and folate. Interestingly, you may think, the juice, fruit and peel of a lime are used to make medicines and help cure severe diarrhea. Limes also kill germs in the skin, aiding in skin care *(preventing aging);* they ease constipation and help prevent fever, urinary tract and bladder infections, ulcers, heart disease *(lowering bad cholesterol)* and even arthritis.

Weight Loss Tip: Drink 4-5 bottles of cold water today.

THE "7" DAY DETOX | THE 21 DAY GREEN-DETOX FAST

BEATS

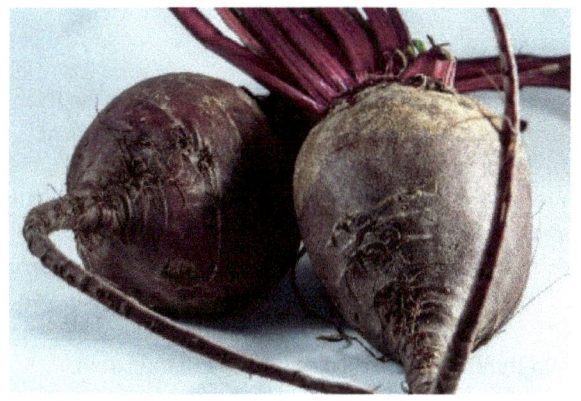

Photo Credit: Digidreamgrafix
Freedigitalphotos.net

WEEK 2, DAY 14
(CARROT BEAT DASHER)

Day 7 of Week 2: Carrot, Beat, 100% Carrot Juice, Parsley, Kale

Add 1 cup of a diced carrot into a blender, Add 1 cup of a diced beat, Add 1/2 cup of 100% Carrot Juice, Add 1/2 cup of parsley, Add 1/2 cup of kale, blend until smooth, pour into a chilled glass or bullet to go blender cup or blender mug, Serve immediately

Health Notes:

Beats – Beats cleanse the body and are a tonic for the liver and purifies the blood as well as prevents many forms of cancer. Beats also help reduce depression, high blood pressure, give energy and are a great source of Fiber, Vitamins A, B & C, beta-carotene, Iron, folic acid *(especially for women that are pregnant along with the Vitamin B and Iron)* as well as Potassium and Magnesium. Beats also help you detoxify your body and boost your stamina and bone strength and help fight Alzheimer's disease and inflammation.

Parsley - Parsley comes from the Mediterranean and is rich in Folic Acid, Vitamins C, K, B-12 and A. Parsley boots your immune system (for healthy bones and teeth and preventing urinary, respiratory and intestinal tract infections, excess gas, asthma, diabetes and kidney stones), helps build strong bones, flushes excess fluid from your kidneys, bladder and body, while helping reduce hair loss, high blood pressure, joint pain, constipation, helps fight illness, cancers *(breast and prostate)* and spleen conditions.

Weight Loss Tip: Drink 4-5 bottles of cold water today.

THE "7" DAY DETOX | THE 21 DAY GREEN-DETOX FAST

WEEK 3
MUSTARD GREENS WEEK

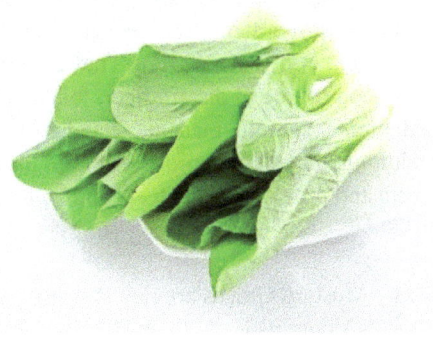

Photo Credit: Mapichai
Freedigitalphotos.net

WEEK 3, DAY 15
(APPLE CARROT LOVER)

Day 1 of Week 3: Apple, Carrot, 100% Vegetable Juice, Mustard Green

Add 1 cup of a diced yellow apple (not green) into a blender, Add 1 cup of a diced carrot, Add 1/2 cup of 100% Vegetable Juice, Add 1/2 cup of mustard greens, blend until smooth, pour into a chilled glass or bullet to go blender cup or blender mug, Serve immediately

Health Notes:

Apples (Yellow) – Apples come in green, yellow and even red. Yellow apples are softer and juicier (sweeter), being that they are rich in Calcium and Water (90%). They are low in calories and are a good source of dietary fiber, folate, niacin, zinc, copper, Vitamin C, thiamin, manganese and even riboflavin. In addition, they help improve memory, maintain urinary tract health and promote strong teeth and bones (green apples).

Mustard Greens – Mustard Greens are rich in many Vitamins and nutrients such as Vitamins K, A, C, E, B-2, B-6, B-1, B-3 and Folate, Iron, Fiber, Copper, Magnesium and Potassium to name a few. Mustard Greens promote a healthy heart, eyes and weight loss. Mustard Greens also aid in detoxifying the body to prevent chronic illnesses *(such as bladder problems, colon, lung, prostate and even ovarian cancers)* because of its rich antioxidant and sulfur-containing nutrients.

Weight Loss Tip: Drink 4-5 bottles of cold water today.

LEMONS

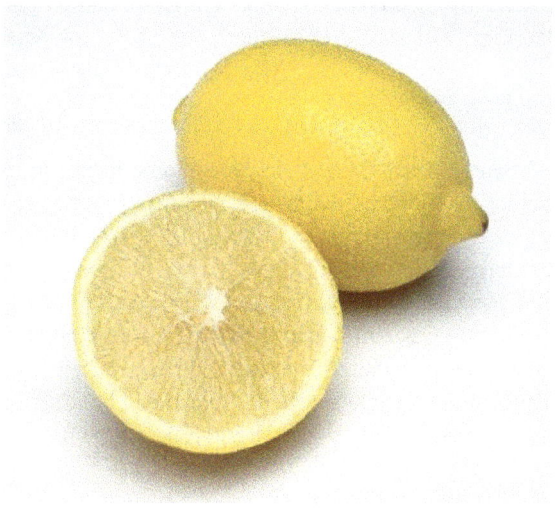

Photo Credit: Suat Eman
Freedigitalphotos.net

WEEK 3, DAY 16
(CARROT BEAT MAKEOVER)

Day 2 of Week 3: Carrot, Beat, dash of squeezed lemon, 100% Vegetable Juice, Parsley, Mustard Green

      Add 1 cup of a diced carrot into a blender, Add 1 cup of a diced beat, Add ½ cup of 100% Vegetable Juice, Add a dash of squeezed lemon, ½ cup of diced parsley, ½ cup of mustard greens, blend until smooth, pour into a chilled glass or bullet to go blender cup or blender mug, Serve immediately

Health Notes:

Beats – Beats cleanse the body and are a tonic for the liver and purifies the blood as well as prevents many forms of cancer. Beats also help reduce depression, high blood pressure, give energy and are a great source of Fiber, Vitamins A, B & C, beta-carotene, Iron, folic acid *(especially for women that are pregnant along with the Vitamin B and Iron)* as well as Potassium and Magnesium. Beats also help you detoxify your body and boost your stamina and bone strength and help fight Alzheimer's disease and inflammation.

Lemons – Lemons are a great source of citric acid, Vitamin C, Calcium and even Potassium. They also help fight hair loss, lumps on the skin and hands, high blood pressure, arthritis, constipation, burns, vision loss, excess gas, gallstones, internal bleeding, fevers and indigestion as well as aids in cleansing the teeth and dandruff from the hair. Lemons also help revitalize your skin and aid in weight loss when mixed with recipes that have water (or ice) and honey in them.

Weight Loss Tip: Drink 4-5 bottles of cold water today.

THE "7" DAY DETOX | THE 21 DAY GREEN-DETOX FAST

PEARS

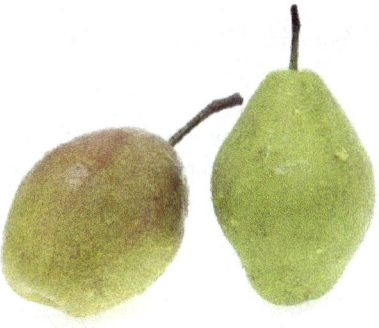

Photo Credit: PhasinPhoto
Freedigitalphotos.net

WEEK 3, DAY 17
(BEAT PEAR LEANER)

Day 3 of Week 3: Beat, Pear, 100% Vegetable Juice, Shot of Wheatgrass, Mustard Green

Add 1 cup of a diced beat into a blender, Add 1 cup of a diced pear, Add 1 small cup of juiced (or non-juiced) wheatgrass, Add 1/2 cup of 100% Vegetable Juice, Add 1/2 cup of mustard greens, blend until smooth, pour into a chilled glass or bullet to go blender cup or blender mug, Serve immediately

Health Notes:

Pears – Pears are filled with Vitamin C and Iron. They are a great source of fiber; help reduce bad cholesterol in the body, fights cancer, acne and aging, increases energy levels and digestion. Pears also help restore shine to your hair and prevents frizz.

Wheatgrass – Wheatgrass is rich in Calcium, Iron, Vitamins A and E and Chlorophyll (helping build the blood). It is also loaded with nutrients and minerals, helping you feel fuller longer and to prevent overeating when you do eat. Wheatgrass also stimulates circulation of oxygen in your body, blood vessels and skin and rids your body of waste. It also helps prevent cancers and tooth decay as well as treats wounds, fatigue, arthritis, sunburn, ulcers (improving digestion), dryness or eczema of the skin (discoloration) and cleanses the skin and liver.

Weight Loss Tip: Drink 4-5 bottles of cold water today.

CARROTS

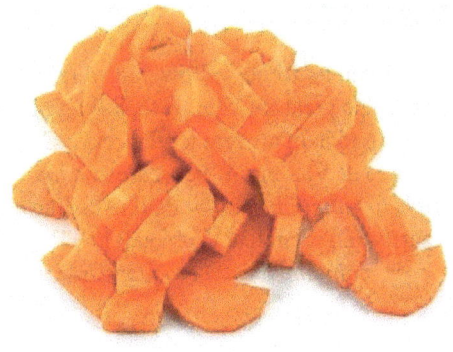

Photo Credit: Grant Cochrane
Freedigitalphotos.net

WEEK 3, DAY 18
(CARROT PRUNER)

Day 4 of Week 3: Carrot, Prune, Mustard Green (in the middle of the week to clean bowels), 100% Vegetable Juice

Add 1 cup of a diced carrot into a blender, Add 1 cup of a diced prune, Add 1/2 cup of 100% Vegetable Juice, Add 1/2 cup of mustard greens, blend until smooth, pour into a chilled glass or bullet to go blender cup or blender mug, Serve immediately

Health Notes:

Carrots - Carrots can be white, yellow, red, purple and orange. They are also great for your teeth, killing off harmful germs in the mouth to help prevent tooth decay. Carrots also have a great source of Vitamin A, beta carotene *(an antioxidant to help maintain healthy skin),* Alkaline elements (which help purify and revitalize the blood) and Potassium *(helping the body maintain normal blood pressure levels).*

Mustard Greens – Mustard Greens are rich in many Vitamins and nutrients such as Vitamins K, A, C, E, B-2, B-6, B-1, B-3 and Folate, Iron, Fiber, Copper, Magnesium and Potassium to name a few. Mustard Greens promote a healthy heart, eyes and weight loss. Mustard Greens also aid in detoxifying the body to prevent chronic illnesses *(such as bladder problems, colon, lung, prostate and even ovarian cancers)* because of its rich antioxidant and sulfur-containing nutrients.

Weight Loss Tip: Drink 4-5 bottles of cold water today.

APPLES

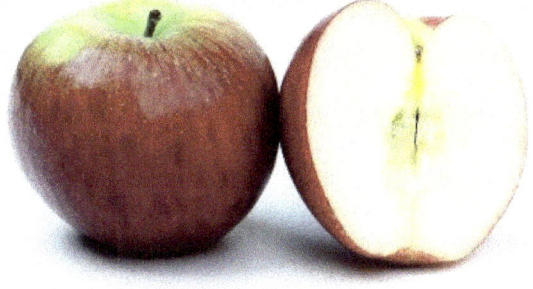

Photo Credit: Paul
Freedigitalphotos.net

WEEK 3, DAY 19
(CUCUMBER APPLE DAISY)

Day 5 of Week 3: Cucumber, Apple, dash of squeezed lemon, 100% Vegetable Juice, Cilantro, Mustard Green

Add 1 cup of a 1/2 diced cucumber into a blender, Add 1 cup of a diced yellow apple (not green), squeezed lemon, Add 1/2 cup of diced Cilantro, Add 1/2 cup of 100% Vegetable Juice, Add 1/2 cup of mustard greens, blend until smooth, pour into a chilled glass or bullet to go blender cup or blender mug, Serve immediately

Health Notes:

Cucumbers – Cucumbers are in the family of melons, squash and pumpkins. They are a great source of Vitamins K, C, A and B and are made up 95% water and are great for the eyes, skin and hair due to their anti-inflammatory properties and hair growth stimulation. They also help fight cancers (ovarian, uterine, breast as well as prostate) and aid in weight loss, digestion, blood pressure control, cholesterol reduction and joint pain relief (that is associated with arthritis). Cucumbers also dissolve kidney stones and rid the body of waste products.

Cilantro – Most people use Cilantro (similar to "dill") in wraps, salads, pastas, pesto, guacamole and even soups. However, really, it can be used in anything. Cilantro is rich in Magnesium, Iron and antioxidants, helping the body fight aging, chronic diseases and food poisoning *(Salmonella; bacteria)*. Due to Cilantros anti-microbial properties and phytonutrients it also helps aid in curing yeast infections, kidney stones and sleep disorders.

Weight Loss Tip: Drink 4-5 bottles of cold water today.

THE "7" DAY DETOX | THE 21 DAY GREEN-DETOX FAST

PINEAPPLES

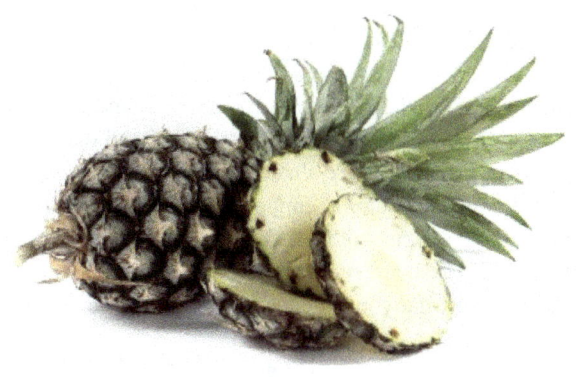

Photo Credit: Rakratchada Torsap
Freedigitalphotos.net

WEEK 3, DAY 20
(PINEAPPLE BEAT CLEANER)
Day 6 of Week 3: Pineapple, Beat, 100% Vegetable Juice, Cilantro, Mustard Green

Add 1 cup of a diced pineapple into a blender, Add 1 cup of a diced beat, Add 1/2 cup of diced Cilantro, Add 1/2 cup of 100% Vegetable Juice, Add 1/2 cup of mustard greens, blend until smooth, pour into a chilled glass or bullet to go blender cup or blender mug, Serve immediately

Health Notes:

Pineapples – Today, the largest producers of pineapples are in Brazil, Costa Rica, the United States, Hawaii and the Philippines. Pineapples are a natural weight loss food and are rich in Vitamin C, Thiamin, copper and boost the immune system to fight against colds, flu symptoms and other diseases. They also help ease arthritis pain, are low in calories and are very filling; keeping you fuller longer, to prevent overeating.

Mustard Greens - Mustard Greens are rich in many Vitamins and nutrients such as Vitamins K, A, C, E, B-2, B-6, B-1, B-3 and Folate, Iron, Fiber, Copper, Magnesium and Potassium to name a few. Mustard Greens promote a healthy heart, eyes and weight loss. Mustard Greens also aid in detoxifying the body to prevent chronic illnesses *(such as bladder problems, colon, lung, prostate and even ovarian cancers)* because of its rich antioxidant and sulfur-containing nutrients.

Weight Loss Tip: Drink 4-5 bottles of cold water today.

CILANTRO

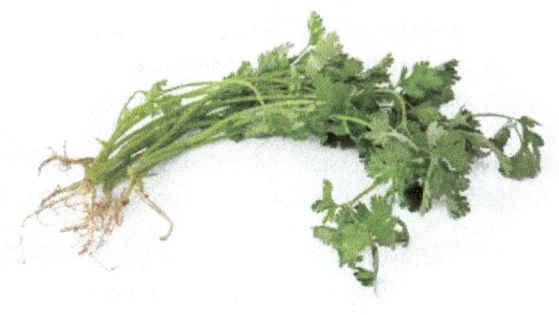

Photo Credit: SOMMAI
Freedigitalphotos.net

WEEK 3, DAY 21
(PEAR CARROT LOVER)

Day 7 of Week 3: Pear, Carrot, 100% Vegetable Juice, Cilantro, Mustard Green

Add 1 cup of a diced pear into a blender, Add 1 cup of a diced carrot, Add a ½ cup of cilantro, Add 1/2 cup of 100% Vegetable Juice, Add 1/2 cup of mustard greens, blend until smooth, pour into a chilled glass or bullet to go blender cup or blender mug, Serve immediately

Health Notes:

Carrots - Carrots can be white, yellow, red, purple and orange. They are also great for your teeth, killing off harmful germs in the mouth to help prevent tooth decay. Carrots also have a great source of Vitamin A, beta carotene *(an antioxidant to help maintain healthy skin),* Alkaline elements (which help purify and revitalize the blood) and Potassium *(helping the body maintain normal blood pressure levels).*

Pears – Pears are filled with Vitamin C and Iron. They are a great source of fiber; help reduce bad cholesterol in the body, fights cancer, acne and aging, increases energy levels and digestion. Pears also help restore shine to your hair and prevents frizz.

Mustard Greens - Mustard Greens are rich in many Vitamins and nutrients such as Vitamins K, A, C, E, B-2, B-6, B-1, B-3 and Folate, Iron, Fiber, Copper, Magnesium and Potassium to name a few. Mustard Greens promote a healthy heart, eyes and weight loss. Mustard Greens also aid in detoxifying the body to prevent chronic illnesses *(such as bladder problems, colon, lung, prostate and even ovarian cancers)* because of its rich antioxidant and sulfur-containing nutrients.

Weight Loss Tip: Drink 4-5 bottles of cold water today.

CONGRATULATIONS ON YOUR NEW YOU!

*Keep up the great work by continuing
on with my two newest books, "The 21 Day Smoothie Fast"
and the "21 Day Salad Fast"*

INDEX OF RECIPES

DAY 1	42		DAY 12	64
DAY 2	44		DAY 13	66
DAY 3	46		DAY 14	68
DAY 4	48		DAY 15	70
DAY 5	50		DAY 16	72
DAY 6	52		DAY 17	74
DAY 7	54		DAY 18	76
DAY 8	56		DAY 19	78
DAY 9	58		DAY 20	80
DAY 10	60		DAY 21	82
DAY 11	62			

THE "7" DAY DETOX | THE 21 DAY GREEN-DETOX FAST

www.ingramcontent.com/pod-product-compliance
Lightning Source LLC
Chambersburg PA
CBHW071841090426
42811CB00035B/2302/J